Yoga and Meditation for Stress Relief

Overcome Anxiety, Improve Sleep Quality, Cultivate Mindfulness, and Achieve a Serene State of Mind

Prem Sagar Sunchu

Copyright © 2024 by Prem Sagar Sunchu

All rights reserved.

No part of this book may be reproduced in any form without permission in writing from the author.

No part of this publication may be reproduced or transmitted in any form or by any means, mechanical or electronic, including photocopying or recording, or by any information storage and retrieval system, or transmitted by email or by any other means whatsoever without permission in writing from the author.

YOUR FREE GIFT !!

As a token of my thanks for taking out time to read my book, I would like to offer you a **Free-Gift**:

Click the Below Link and Download your **Free eBook PDF**.

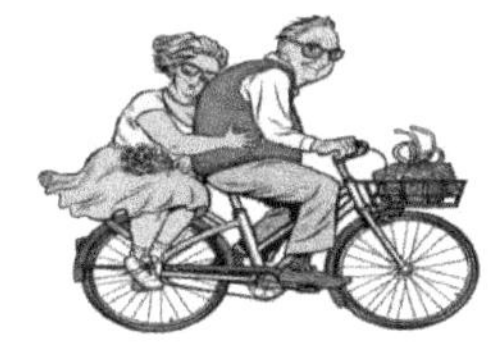

"The Joyful Tapestry: A Global Mission for Happiness"

Or **Scan the QR Code** Below:

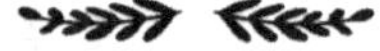

ABOUT THE AUTHOR

Prem Sagar Sunchu, the Accomplished Author of "Yoga and Meditation for Stress Relief"

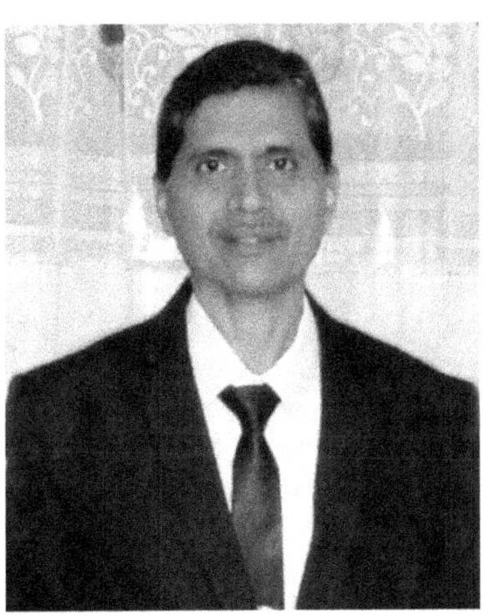

Meet Mr. Prem Sagar, an ordinary soul born in the vibrant city of Secunderabad, India, where the tapestry of life weaves stories of resilience and dreams. His journey is a testament to the power of perpetual learning, where every encounter is a lesson, and every moment holds the potential for growth.

A man of many dimensions, Mr. Sagar embodies the qualities of a perpetual student, a dedicated listener, and a dreamer who gazes at the stars but keeps his feet firmly grounded. His aspirations soar high, and his relentless pursuit of them is fueled by a genuine desire to make a positive impact on those around him.

Having served as a Chief Manager in the prestigious State Bank of India, Mr. Sagar brings a wealth of experience from the world of banking. However, for him, retirement isn't a conclusion but a commencement—a reminder that life's true journey begins when one can reflect on the wisdom gained from the first innings.

In Mr. Sagar's view, retirement is not a retreat but a stepping stone to a realm of infinite possibilities. It's an opportunity to surpass the ordinary, where the canvas of life awaits new brushstrokes of creativity and purpose. For him, the "be good and do good policy" isn't just a mantra; it's a guiding principle that shapes his approach to life.

As he embraces the second innings, Mr. Sagar encourages others to view retirement not as a winding down but as a springboard to new endeavors. It's a time when accumulated wisdom meets fresh energy, and the monotony of routine gives way to the vibrancy of creativity. His belief is clear: retirement is not just a number; it's a chapter where the richness of experience meets the possibilities in abundance.

In the world of Mr. Prem Sagar, retirement is not a period of rest but a canvas waiting to be painted with the colors of newfound wisdom, creativity, and a different outlook on life.

Prem Sagar Sunchu
M.Com, LLM, Certified Independent Director (IICA)
GOI,
Author, Sole Arbitrator and Legal Consultant, Freelancer

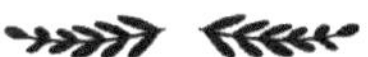

ACKNOWLEDGEMENTS

In profound gratitude, I extend heartfelt appreciation to my amazing parents. To my caring and resilient mother, **Smt. S.L. Lakshmi**, who gracefully navigated the challenges of my father's service transfers, made countless sacrifices to bind our family together. My father, **Shri S.R. Lakshman Rao**, stands as my enduring role model—his post-retirement vibrancy, marked by a dedicated hobby of reading and writing, serves as the very foundation that propels me into the realm of authorship.

A debt of gratitude is owed to my beautiful wife, **Smt. S.P. Padma Sree** is a constant source of inspiration, unwavering strength, and invaluable guidance. Balancing family responsibilities and the intricate path of an author, her presence has been the foundation of my journey.

To my handsome sons, **S.P. Gautam Sagar, S.P. Prayag Sagar**, and **S.P. Akshaj Sagar**, whose unwavering support and responsibility bear testament to the great strength they provide. Their motivation fuels my endeavors across all the diverse traits I undertake.

I owe thanks to **Mr. Som Bathla**, an **Amazon #1 Best-selling** author, for his mentorship, motivation, and guidance in the realms of **Writing, Self-Publishing, and Launching Books**. His support has been instrumental in initiating my journey as an Authorpreneur.

My Sincere thanks to **Mr. Sooraj Achar**, who is also an Amazon Bestselling Author, for his **Professional Editing,** Formatting, and Publishing support.

In acknowledging these pillars of support, I am reminded that the tapestry of my life and authorial pursuit is woven with threads of love, sacrifice, and inspiration. With profound thanks to my family, who stand as my bedrock of strength and motivation.

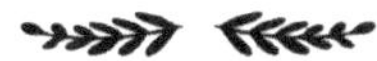

To the guiding stars of my universe—my Parents, Grand-parents, Parents-in-law, Brothers, Sisters, the cherished members of our extended Family and Friends. Their un-wavering support and boundless encouragement have been the driving force behind my Author Journey.

In the tapestry of my life, each of them has woven threads of inspiration and resilience, transforming mere words into stories and dreams into realities. Their confidence in me has been a constant source of strength, propelling me forward through the path of this journey.

With heartfelt gratitude, I dedicate the pages of my work to the pillars of love and encouragement that they are, rec-ognizing that every word I pen is a tribute to the collective spirit of our family. May this dedication reflect the depth of my appreciation for the profound impact they have had on my creative journey.

"Yoga and Meditation for Stress Relief" is my second book in the series of five books-**"Holistic Well-being: A Journey to Balance"**

Contents

INTRODUCTION

Welcome to Your Journey of Serenity

In our fast-paced, modern world, stress has become an almost unavoidable companion. It infiltrates our daily lives, often leaving us feeling overwhelmed, anxious, and disconnected from our true selves. While some stress can be beneficial, propelling us towards growth and achievement, chronic stress can be debilitating, leading to a host of physical, emotional, and mental health issues. But what if there was a way to reclaim your peace, enhance your well-being, and transform stress into a tool for personal growth and mindfulness?

Welcome to "Yoga and Meditation for Stress Relief," a comprehensive guide designed to help you overcome anxiety, improve sleep quality, cultivate mindfulness, and achieve a serene state of mind. This book is not just a collection of techniques; it's a roadmap to a more balanced, harmonious life. Whether you are a beginner looking to dip your toes into the world of yoga and meditation or an experienced practitioner seeking to deepen your practice, this book offers valuable insights and practical tools to support your journey.

The Essence of Yoga and Meditation

Yoga and meditation are ancient practices that have been embraced by millions worldwide for their profound benefits on the mind, body, and spirit. At their core, both practices are about cultivating awareness and harmony within ourselves and with the world around us. Yoga, with its physical postures (asanas), breath control (pranayama), and ethical principles, prepares the body and mind for deeper states of meditation. Meditation, in turn, helps to calm the mind, reduce stress, and foster a deeper sense of inner peace and clarity.

Why Focus on Stress Relief?

The impact of stress on our lives cannot be overstated. From insomnia and anxiety to chronic illnesses and mental health disorders, the consequences of unmanaged stress are far-reaching. Understanding stress and learning how to manage it effectively can lead to a dramatic improvement in your overall quality of life. This book aims to equip you with the knowledge and tools necessary to combat stress through the powerful practices of yoga and meditation.

What You Will Learn

In this book, you will embark on a transformative journey through carefully structured chapters that build upon each other to provide a holistic approach to stress relief:

1. Understanding Stress and Its Impact: Gain a deep understanding of what stress is, how it affects your body and mind, and why it's crucial to manage it effectively.

2. The Fundamentals of Yoga for Stress Relief: Learn the basics of yoga, including key postures and breathing techniques that specifically target stress reduction.

3. Exploring Meditation Techniques: Discover various meditation practices, from mindfulness to guided imagery, and find the methods that work best for you.

4. Creating a Holistic Stress Relief Plan: Integrate yoga, meditation, and lifestyle changes into a cohesive plan tailored to your unique needs and circumstances.

5. Advanced Yoga and Meditation Practices: Take your practice to the next level with advanced techniques designed to deepen your relaxation and mindfulness.

6. Long-Term Stress Relief Strategies: Develop sustainable habits and strategies that will help you maintain a serene state of mind and a balanced lifestyle over the long term.

Embark on Your Path to Serenity

This book is your companion on the path to a calmer, more centered life. Each chapter is designed to guide you step-by-step, offering practical advice, detailed instructions, and inspirational insights. By the end of this journey, you will have developed a personalized toolkit of yoga and meditation practices that empower you to handle stress with grace and ease.

Prepare to transform your relationship with stress, enhance your well-being, and discover a deeper sense of peace and contentment. Your journey to a serene state of mind begins now. Let's embark on this path together, one mindful breath at a time.

Chapter 1

Understanding Stress and Its Impact

"In times of stress, the best thing we can do for each other is to listen with our ears and our hearts and to be assured that our questions are just as important as our answers." – Fred Rogers

Introduction

Stress is an inevitable part of modern life. Whether it's related to work, relationships, health, or the myriad demands of daily living, stress affects everyone at some point. While a certain amount of stress can be beneficial, serving as a motivator and helping us to respond to challenges, chronic stress can have profound negative effects on both our physical and mental well-being. This chapter delves into the nature of stress, its impacts, and various approaches to managing it, including the time-honored practices of yoga and meditation.

1.1 The Science of Stress

Stress is the body's response to perceived threats or challenges, triggering a cascade of physiological and psychological reactions. At its core, stress is an evolutionary mechanism designed to help organisms cope with danger. When faced with a stressor, the body initiates the "fight or flight" response, releasing hormones like adrenaline and cortisol.

These hormones prepare the body for immediate action: the heart rate increases, blood pressure rises, and energy is diverted from non-essential functions to the muscles. While this response is crucial in life-threatening situations, modern stressors are often chronic and psychological, such as job pressure or financial worries, leading to prolonged activation of this stress response and resulting in adverse health outcomes.

Research has shown that chronic stress can lead to numerous health issues, including cardiovascular diseases, weakened immune function, digestive problems, and mental health disorders like anxiety and depression. Understanding the science of stress is the first step towards managing its impact and improving overall well-being.

1.2 How Stress Affects the Body and Mind

The effects of stress on the body and mind are extensive and interrelated. Physically, chronic stress can manifest in various ways. Cardiovascular problems, such as hypertension and heart disease, are common in individuals experiencing long-term stress. This is due to the continuous strain placed on the heart and blood vessels by stress hormones.

The immune system is another casualty of chronic stress. Prolonged exposure to stress hormones can suppress the immune response, making the body more susceptible to infections and diseases. Stress also impacts digestive health, often exacerbating conditions like irritable bowel syndrome (IBS) and gastritis.

Mentally, stress can lead to conditions such as anxiety, depression, and cognitive impairments. The constant state of alertness and worry drains mental resources, leading to difficulties in concentration, memory issues, and a general sense of mental fatigue. Furthermore, stress can disrupt sleep patterns, contributing to a cycle of insomnia and further cognitive decline.

Emotional well-being is also compromised under chronic stress. Individuals may experience mood swings, irritability, and a sense of helplessness. These emotional states can strain personal relationships and reduce overall quality of life.

1.3 Traditional and Modern Approaches to Stress Management

Managing stress is a multi-faceted endeavor that combines traditional practices with modern techniques. Traditional approaches to stress management often include physical activities, dietary adjustments, and herbal remedies.

Physical activity, such as walking, swimming, or engaging in sports, has been a long-standing method to alleviate stress. Exercise stimulates the production of endorphins, which are natural mood lifters. Dietary changes, including the incorporation of foods rich in omega-3 fatty acids, antioxidants, and magnesium, can also help mitigate stress.

Herbal remedies like chamomile, lavender, and valerian root have been used for centuries to promote relaxation and reduce anxiety. These natural treatments are still popular today, often in the form of teas, supplements, or essential oils.

Modern stress management techniques include cognitive-behavioral therapy (CBT), mindfulness-based stress reduction (MBSR), and various relaxation techniques. CBT helps individuals identify and change negative thought patterns that contribute to stress, while MBSR focuses on cultivating present-moment awareness and acceptance.

Relaxation techniques, such as deep breathing exercises, progressive muscle relaxation, and guided imagery, are effective tools for reducing stress. These methods help calm the mind and body, breaking the cycle of chronic stress.

1.4 Introduction to Yoga

Yoga, an ancient practice originating in India, has gained widespread popularity as a holistic approach to stress management. Combining physical postures (asanas), breathing exercises (pranayama), and meditation (dhyana), yoga offers a comprehensive system for promoting physical, mental, and emotional well-being.

The physical aspect of yoga involves a series of postures that stretch, strengthen, and relax the muscles. These movements enhance flexibility, improve circulation, and promote the release of tension stored in the body. Regular practice of yoga asanas has been shown to lower blood pressure, improve heart health, and boost immune function.

Breathing exercises in yoga, known as pranayama, are designed to regulate the flow of vital energy (prana) in the body. Techniques such as deep diaphragmatic breathing, alternate nostril breathing, and breath retention can help calm the nervous system, reduce anxiety, and increase mental clarity.

Meditation is a core component of yoga, focusing on mindfulness and inner peace. Through meditation, practitioners learn to observe their thoughts without judgment, fostering a sense of detachment and reducing the impact of stressors. Meditation also enhances concentration, emotional resilience, and overall mental health.

Yoga's emphasis on the mind-body connection makes it a powerful tool for stress management. By integrating physical movement, breath control, and meditation, yoga addresses stress holistically, promoting harmony and balance.

1.5 Introduction to Meditation

Meditation is a practice that involves focusing the mind and eliminating distractions to achieve a state of mental clarity and emotional calm. It has been practiced for thousands of years in various cultural and religious traditions, and its benefits for stress reduction are well-documented.

There are many forms of meditation, but they all share the common goal of quieting the mind. Mindfulness meditation, for example, involves paying attention to the present moment without judgment. Practitioners focus on their breath, bodily sensations, or a specific object, allowing thoughts to come and go without attachment.

Another popular form is transcendental meditation, which uses the repetition of a mantra to help practitioners achieve a deep state of relaxation and heightened awareness. This form of meditation is particularly effective in reducing stress and anxiety.

Loving-kindness meditation, or Metta, involves directing feelings of love and compassion towards oneself and others. This practice fosters positive emotions and reduces feelings of stress and negativity.

Research has shown that regular meditation practice can reduce the levels of stress hormones in the body, improve immune function, and increase the size of brain regions associated with emotional regulation and self-control. Meditation also enhances attention, memory, and overall cognitive function.

Incorporating meditation into daily life can provide a powerful buffer against the stresses of modern living. By fostering a sense of inner peace and resilience, meditation helps individuals navigate life's challenges with greater ease and equanimity.

Conclusion

Understanding stress and its impact is crucial for maintaining a healthy and balanced life. The science of stress reveals how chronic stress can detrimentally affect both the body and mind, leading to a range of health issues. Traditional and modern approaches to stress management offer valuable tools for alleviating stress and promoting well-being. Among these, yoga and meditation stand out as particularly effective practices, addressing stress holistically and fostering a sense of harmony and peace. By integrating these practices into daily life, individuals can cultivate resilience and improve their overall quality of life.

Resources

1. Books:

- Sapolsky, R. M. (2004). Why Zebras Don't Get Ulcers: The Acclaimed Guide to Stress, Stress-Related Diseases, and Coping.

- Kabat-Zinn, J. (1990). Full Catastrophe Living: Using the Wisdom of Your Body and Mind to Face Stress, Pain, and Illness.

2. Articles:

- McEwen, B. S. (2007). "Physiology and Neurobiology of Stress and Adaptation: Central Role of the Brain." Physiological Reviews, 87(3), 873-904.

- Hoffman, J. W., et al. (1982). "Psychosocial Influences on Upper Respiratory Infectious Disease in a Controlled Environment." Psychosomatic Medicine, 44(6), 493-497.

3. Websites:

- American Psychological Association. (2021). "Stress Management." [apa.org](https://www.apa.org/topics/stress)

- Mayo Clinic. (2021). "Stress Management." [mayoclinic.org](https://www.mayoclinic.org/healthy-lifestyle/stress-management/basics/stress-basics/hlv-20049495)

4. Meditation Apps:

- Headspace: [headspace.com](https://www.headspace.com)

- Calm: [calm.com](https://www.calm.com)

These resources provide a comprehensive foundation for further exploration of stress management techniques and the benefits of yoga and meditation.

CHAPTER 2

THE FUNDAMENTALS OF YOGA FOR STRESS RELIEF

"Yoga is not about touching your toes, it's about what you learn on the way down." – Jigar Gor

Introduction

Yoga, an ancient practice with origins in India, has been celebrated for its holistic approach to health and well-being. In recent decades, it has gained widespread popularity worldwide as an effective tool for stress relief. By integrating physical postures, breath control, and meditation, yoga offers a multifaceted approach to managing stress and promoting overall wellness. This chapter explores the fundamentals of yoga for stress relief, providing readers with essential knowledge and practical guidance to begin or deepen their yoga practice.

2.1 Basic Yoga Poses for Beginners

Starting a yoga practice can be both exciting and intimidating for beginners. However, understanding and practicing a few fundamental poses can provide a solid foundation and boost confidence. These poses not only enhance physical strength and flexibility but also promote relaxation and stress reduction.

Mountain Pose (Tadasana)

Mountain Pose is a foundational standing pose that promotes grounding and stability. It involves standing tall with feet hip-width apart, arms at the sides, and palms facing forward. This pose helps improve posture, balance, and body awareness.

Child's Pose (Balasana)

Child's Pose is a gentle resting pose that calms the mind and relieves tension in the back, shoulders, and neck. From a kneeling position, sit back on the heels, stretch the arms forward, and rest the forehead on the mat. This pose encourages deep breathing and relaxation.

Cat-Cow Pose (Marjaryasana-Bitilasana)

Cat-Cow Pose is a flowing sequence that enhances flexibility in the spine and promotes mindful movement. Begin on hands and knees, with wrists aligned under shoulders and knees under hips. Inhale, arch the back (Cow Pose), and exhale, round the spine (Cat Pose). This sequence warms up the spine and encourages a connection between breath and movement.

Downward-Facing Dog (Adho Mukha Svanasana)

Downward-Facing Dog is a widely recognized pose that stretches the entire body, particularly the hamstrings, calves, and shoulders. From a hands-and-knees position, lift the hips upward, forming an inverted V-shape. This pose increases blood flow to the brain and energizes the body.

Standing Forward Bend (Uttanasana)

Standing Forward Bend is a calming pose that stretches the hamstrings, calves, and lower back. From a standing position, hinge at the hips and fold forward, letting the head and arms hang. This pose promotes relaxation and reduces stress by encouraging the release of tension in the upper body.

Corpse Pose (Savasana)

Corpse Pose is typically practiced at the end of a yoga session to facilitate deep relaxation. Lie flat on the back with arms at the sides, palms facing up, and legs comfortably apart. Close the eyes and focus on deep, slow breathing. This pose helps integrate the benefits of the practice and induces a state of restful awareness.

2.2 Breath Control and Pranayama

Breath control, or pranayama, is a fundamental aspect of yoga that involves regulating the breath to enhance physical and mental well-being. Pranayama techniques can calm the nervous system, reduce stress, and improve overall health.

Diaphragmatic Breathing (Deep Belly Breathing)

Diaphragmatic breathing, also known as deep belly breathing, involves breathing deeply into the abdomen rather than shallowly into the chest. This technique activates the body's relaxation response, lowers heart rate, and reduces stress. To practice, sit or lie down comfortably, place one hand on the chest and the other on the abdomen. Inhale deeply through the nose, allowing the abdomen to rise, and exhale slowly through the mouth, letting the abdomen fall.

Nadi Shodhana (Alternate Nostril Breathing)

Nadi Shodhana, or alternate nostril breathing, balances the left and right hemispheres of the brain and calms the mind. To practice, sit comfortably and use the right thumb to close the right nostril. Inhale deeply through the left nostril, then close the left nostril with the ring finger and exhale through the right nostril. Continue this pattern, alternating nostrils with each breath.

Ujjayi Breath (Ocean Breath)

Ujjayi breath, also known as ocean breath, involves constricting the throat slightly to create a soft, whispering sound during inhalation and exhalation. This breath technique promotes focus and relaxation during yoga practice. To practice, inhale and exhale through the nose while gently constricting the back of the throat, creating a sound reminiscent of ocean waves.

Bhramari (Bee Breath)

Bhramari, or bee breath, involves humming to create soothing vibrations that calm the nervous system. To practice, sit comfortably, close the eyes, and take a deep breath in. On the exhale, hum like a bee, focusing on the vibrations in the head and throat. This technique can reduce anxiety and promote relaxation.

Kapalabhati (Skull Shining Breath)

Kapalabhati, or skull shining breath, is an energizing pranayama technique that involves rapid, forceful exhalations followed by passive inhalations. This technique clears the mind and invigorates the body. To practice, sit comfortably, take a deep breath in, and then exhale forcefully through the nose, pulling the navel toward the spine. Allow passive inhalation and continue the cycle.

2.3 Developing a Consistent Yoga Practice

Consistency is key to reaping the benefits of yoga for stress relief. Establishing a regular practice can help integrate yoga into daily life and foster long-term well-being.

Setting Realistic Goals

Setting realistic goals is crucial for developing a sustainable yoga practice. Begin by identifying specific objectives, such as improving flexibility, reducing stress, or enhancing mindfulness. Start with short, manageable sessions, and gradually increase the duration and complexity as comfort and confidence grow.

Creating a Dedicated Space

Creating a dedicated space for yoga practice can enhance focus and motivation. Choose a quiet, clutter-free area with enough room to move freely. Consider adding elements that promote relaxation, such as candles, incense, or calming music.

Establishing a Routine

Establishing a routine helps make yoga a regular part of daily life. Choose a consistent time each day to practice, whether it's in the morning to energize the body or in the evening to unwind. Consistency in timing reinforces the habit and makes it easier to maintain a regular practice.

Incorporating Variety

Incorporating variety into yoga practice can prevent boredom and keep motivation high. Explore different styles of yoga, such as Hatha, Vinyasa, or Yin, and try new poses or sequences. Additionally, attending yoga classes or following online tutorials can provide fresh inspiration and guidance.

Listening to the Body

Listening to the body is essential for a safe and effective yoga practice. Pay attention to physical sensations and avoid pushing beyond comfortable limits. Modify poses as needed and take breaks when necessary. Respecting the body's signals helps prevent injury and promotes a more enjoyable practice.

Tracking Progress

Tracking progress can boost motivation and provide a sense of accomplishment. Keep a journal to record practice sessions, noting any challenges, achievements, and changes in physical or mental well-being. Reflecting on progress can highlight the benefits of yoga and encourage continued practice.

2.4 Yoga for Specific Stress-Related Issues

Yoga can be tailored to address specific stress-related issues, providing targeted relief and enhancing overall well-being.

Yoga for Anxiety

Anxiety often involves excessive worry and a heightened state of alertness. Yoga poses that promote relaxation and grounding can help alleviate anxiety symptoms. Poses such as Child's Pose, Legs Up the Wall, and Corpse Pose encourage relaxation and reduce tension. Additionally, pranayama techniques like Nadi Shodhana and Bhramari can calm the nervous system and ease anxious thoughts.

Yoga for Depression

Depression is characterized by persistent feelings of sadness and low energy. Yoga can help lift the mood and increase energy levels. Poses that open the chest, such as Cobra Pose and Bridge Pose, can counteract the hunched posture often associated with depression and stimulate the flow of energy. Sun Salutations, a sequence of flowing movements, can invigorate the body and mind.

Yoga for Insomnia

Insomnia involves difficulty falling or staying asleep. Yoga poses that promote relaxation and prepare the body for rest can improve sleep quality. Poses such as Forward Bend, Reclining Bound Angle Pose, and Corpse Pose can calm the mind and body. Pranayama techniques like Diaphragmatic Breathing and Ujjayi Breath can also induce a state of relaxation conducive to sleep.

Yoga for Chronic Pain

Chronic pain can lead to physical and emotional stress. Gentle yoga poses that enhance flexibility and reduce tension can alleviate pain and promote well-being. Poses such as Cat-Cow, Child's Pose, and Pigeon Pose can stretch and relax tight muscles. Mindfulness meditation and pranayama can also help manage pain by shifting focus and promoting relaxation.

Yoga for Fatigue

Fatigue involves a persistent feeling of tiredness and lack of energy. Yoga poses that stimulate and energize the body can counteract fatigue. Poses such as Downward-Facing Dog, Warrior II, and Tree Pose can increase circulation and vitality. Incorporating breathwork, like Kapalabhati, can also invigorate the body and mind.

2.5 Restorative Yoga for Deep Relaxation

Restorative yoga is a gentle, supportive practice that focuses on deep relaxation and stress relief. It involves holding poses for extended periods, often with the support of props like blankets, bolsters, and blocks.

Supported Child's Pose

Supported Child's Pose provides a deeply relaxing stretch for the back and hips. Use a bolster or stack of blankets to support the torso and allow the body

Resources

To deepen your understanding and practice of yoga for stress relief, consider exploring the following books, articles, videos, and online resources:

Books

1. "The Heart of Yoga: Developing a Personal Practice" by T.K.V. Desikachar

- This book offers a comprehensive guide to the principles and practice of yoga, making it accessible to practitioners of all levels.

2. "Light on Yoga" by B.K.S. Iyengar

- A classic in the field, this book provides detailed instructions and illustrations for numerous yoga poses, along with insights into the philosophy of yoga.

3. "Yoga for Stress Relief: A Simple and Unique Three-Month Yoga Program for Your Body, Mind, and Spirit" by Swami Saradananda

- This practical guide presents a structured program for using yoga to manage and alleviate stress.

4. "The Relaxation and Stress Reduction Workbook" by Martha Davis, Elizabeth Robbins Eshelman, and Matthew McKay

- While not exclusively about yoga, this workbook includes yoga-based techniques alongside other methods for reducing stress.

5. "The Yoga Sutras of Patanjali" translated by Sri Swami Satchidananda

- This ancient text is fundamental to understanding the philosophy and deeper aspects of yoga practice.

Articles and Journals

1. "Yoga as an Intervention for Psychological and Physiological Health" by Holger Cramer, Romy Lauche, et al.

- Published in Frontiers in Psychiatry, this review article explores the evidence supporting yoga's benefits for mental and physical health.

2. "Effects of Yoga on Mental and Physical Health: A Short Summary of Reviews" by Holger Cramer, Romy Lauche, et al.

- Published in Evidence-Based Complementary and Alternative Medicine, this article summarizes research findings on yoga's health benefits.

3. "Yoga for Anxiety and Depression" by P. L. Streeter, S. M. Gerbarg, et al.

- Published in Harvard Review of Psychiatry, this article reviews the effectiveness of yoga as a treatment for anxiety and depression.

4. "The Effectiveness of Yoga for Depression: A Critical Literature Review" by Ying Chen, Catherine E. Yang, et al.

- Published in The Journal of Clinical Psychiatry, this review examines the impact of yoga on depression symptoms.

5. "Impact of Yoga on the Brain: A Review of Current Research" by Rael Cahn and Julian Polich

- Published in Frontiers in Human Neuroscience, this article discusses the neurological effects of yoga practice.

Videos

1. "Yoga with Adriene" (YouTube Channel)

- Adriene Mishler offers a variety of yoga videos, including sessions specifically for stress relief, beginners, and restorative practices.

- [Yoga with Adriene](https://www.youtube.com/user/yogawithadriene)

2. "Yoga Journal" (YouTube Channel)

- This channel provides instructional videos on various yoga poses, sequences, and pranayama techniques.

- [Yoga Journal](https://www.youtube.com/user/yogajournal)

3. "Tara Stiles Yoga" (YouTube Channel)

- Tara Stiles shares approachable yoga routines, including practices aimed at reducing stress and promoting relaxation.

- [Tara Stiles Yoga](https://www.youtube.com/user/TaraStilesYoga)

Online Resources

1. Yoga Alliance

- The Yoga Alliance website offers resources for finding certified yoga instructors, online classes, and educational materials.

- [Yoga Alliance](https://www.yogaalliance.org)

2. DoYogaWithMe

- This website provides free online yoga classes for all levels, including specific programs for stress relief and relaxation.

- [DoYogaWithMe](https://www.doyogawithme.com)

3. Gaia

- Gaia offers a subscription service with access to a vast library of yoga videos, including sessions focused on stress management and mindfulness.

- [Gaia](https://www.gaia.com)

4. Yoga International

- This platform offers articles, videos, and courses on various aspects of yoga, including therapeutic yoga for stress and anxiety.

- [Yoga International](https://yogainternational.com)

5. Mindful

- While not exclusively about yoga, Mindful provides resources on mindfulness practices that complement yoga, including articles, guided meditations, and online courses.

- [Mindful](https://www.mindful.org)

Apps

1. Yoga Studio: Mind & Body

- This app offers pre-made and customizable yoga classes, including options for stress relief and relaxation.

- Available on [iOS] (https://apps.apple.com/us/app/yoga-studio-mind-body/id567767430) and [Android] (https://play.google.com/store/apps/details?id=com.gaiam.yogastudio).

2. Headspace

- While primarily a meditation app, Headspace includes yoga and movement sessions designed to reduce stress and promote relaxation.

- Available on [iOS] (https://apps.apple.com/us/app/headspace-meditation-sleep/id493145008) and [Android] (https://play.google.com/store/apps/details?id=com.getsomeheadspace.android).

3. Daily Yoga

- Daily Yoga offers guided yoga sessions for all levels, with specific programs for stress relief and emotional well-being.

- Available on [iOS] (https://apps.apple.com/us/a
pp/daily-yoga-workout-fitness/id545849922) and [An-
droid] (https://play.google.com/store/apps/details?id=co
m.dailyyoga.inc).

By leveraging these resources, readers can enhance their understanding and practice of yoga for stress relief, fostering a
more balanced and peaceful life.

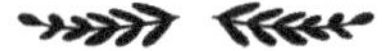

Chapter 3

Exploring Meditation Techniques

"Meditation is not evasion; it is a serene encounter with reality." – Thích Nhất Hạnh

Introduction

Meditation is an ancient practice that transcends cultural and religious boundaries, offering a profound method for achieving mental clarity, emotional balance, and stress relief. This chapter delves into various meditation techniques, each with its unique approach to calming the mind and fostering inner peace. By exploring these techniques, readers can discover which methods resonate most with their personal needs and lifestyles, thereby enhancing their journey toward holistic well-being.

3.1 Mindfulness Meditation

Mindfulness meditation, rooted in Buddhist traditions, has gained widespread recognition for its effectiveness in reducing stress and enhancing mental well-being. This practice involves maintaining a non-judgmental awareness of the present moment, observing thoughts, sensations, and emotions as they arise without attachment.

The Practice of Mindfulness Meditation

To practice mindfulness meditation, find a quiet, comfortable place to sit. Close your eyes and bring your attention to your breath, noticing the sensation of each inhale and exhale. When your mind wanders, gently redirect your focus back to your breath. The goal is not to eliminate thoughts but to observe them without getting caught up in them.

Benefits of Mindfulness Meditation

Research has shown that mindfulness meditation can significantly reduce symptoms of anxiety, depression, and chronic pain. It enhances emotional regulation, improves focus, and promotes a greater sense of overall well-being. Studies have also indicated that regular mindfulness practice can lead to structural changes in the brain, increasing grey matter density in areas associated with memory, learning, and emotional regulation.

3.2 Focused Attention Meditation

Focused attention meditation, also known as concentrative meditation, involves directing all of your attention to a single point of focus, such as the breath, a mantra, or a visual object. This practice helps develop concentration and mental clarity by training the mind to remain steady on one point.

The Practice of Focused Attention Meditation

Choose a point of focus for your meditation, such as your breath. Sit comfortably and close your eyes. Concentrate on your chosen focus, and when distractions arise, gently bring your attention back. Common focuses include a mantra, a candle flame, or the sensation of the breath at the nostrils.

Benefits of Focused Attention Meditation

Focused attention meditation enhances the ability to concentrate and reduces the mind's tendency to wander. It can improve cognitive performance, reduce stress, and foster a sense of inner calm. Regular practice can also increase attention span and mental resilience, making it easier to handle daily challenges with a clear and focused mind.

3.3 Loving-Kindness Meditation

Loving-kindness meditation, or Metta meditation, is a practice that cultivates unconditional love and compassion towards oneself and others. This technique involves silently repeating phrases that express goodwill and kindness, initially directing them towards oneself and gradually extending them to others, including loved ones, acquaintances, and even difficult individuals.

The Practice of Loving-Kindness Meditation

Begin by sitting comfortably with your eyes closed. Take a few deep breaths and bring to mind a sense of warmth and compassion. Silently repeat phrases such as "May I be happy, may I be healthy, may I be safe, may I live with ease." After a few minutes, direct these phrases towards others, starting with someone you care about, then a neutral person, and finally someone with whom you have difficulties.

Benefits of Loving-Kindness Meditation

Loving-kindness meditation enhances positive emotions, reduces negative emotional states, and increases empathy and compassion. Research has shown that this practice can lead to improvements in emotional well-being and resilience, reduce symptoms of anxiety and depression, and even positively affect physical health by lowering stress-related inflammation and enhancing immune function.

3.4 Body Scan Meditation

Body scan meditation is a mindfulness practice that involves systematically focusing attention on different parts of the body, promoting awareness and relaxation. This technique helps to release physical tension and fosters a deep connection between mind and body.

The Practice of Body Scan Meditation

Lie down comfortably on your back with your eyes closed. Begin by taking a few deep breaths, then direct your attention to your toes, noticing any sensations without trying to change them. Gradually move your attention up through the body, from the feet to the head, observing sensations in each area. If you notice tension, acknowledge it without judgment and move on.

Benefits of Body Scan Meditation

Body scan meditation can reduce stress and physical tension, enhance body awareness, and improve sleep quality. It encourages relaxation and helps in identifying areas of chronic tension that may be contributing to stress. Studies suggest that regular practice can lower levels of cortisol, the stress hormone, and improve overall emotional regulation.

3.5 Guided Imagery and Visualization

Guided imagery and visualization involve using mental images to promote relaxation, healing, and positive thinking. This technique can be self-directed or led by a guide, often incorporating narratives that evoke calming or uplifting images.

The Practice of Guided Imagery and Visualization

Find a quiet place to sit or lie down comfortably. Close your eyes and take a few deep breaths to relax. Begin to visualize a peaceful scene, such as a beach, forest, or mountain. Engage all your senses in the imagery, noticing the sights, sounds, smells, and tactile sensations. Alternatively, follow a guided session available through apps or online resources that lead you through specific visualizations for relaxation or goal achievement.

Benefits of Guided Imagery and Visualization

Guided imagery and visualization can significantly reduce stress and anxiety, improve mood, and enhance overall well-being. This practice has been shown to lower blood pressure, reduce pain, and boost the immune system. Visualization techniques are also used to enhance performance in various fields, from sports to public speaking, by fostering a positive mindset and increasing confidence.

Conclusion

Meditation offers a diverse array of techniques that cater to different needs and preferences, making it a versatile tool for stress relief and personal growth. From the mindfulness of simply observing the present moment to the compassion cultivated in loving-kindness meditation, each practice has unique benefits that contribute to mental and emotional well-being. By exploring and integrating these meditation techniques, individuals can develop a personalized practice that supports their journey towards inner peace and resilience in the face of life's challenges.

Resources

To further explore and deepen your meditation practice, the following resources provide valuable guidance and support:

Books

1. "The Miracle of Mindfulness" by Thích Nhất Hạnh

- A practical guide to mindfulness meditation, offering techniques and insights from a renowned Zen master.

2. "Wherever You Go, There You Are" by Jon Kabat-Zinn

- An accessible introduction to mindfulness meditation, emphasizing the practice of being present in everyday life.

3. "Lovingkindness: The Revolutionary Art of Happiness" by Sharon Salzberg

- A comprehensive guide to loving-kindness meditation, exploring its principles and practice.

4. "The Body Scan Meditation" by Jon Kabat-Zinn

- A detailed exploration of body scan meditation, its benefits, and its applications in stress reduction and healing.

5. "The Relaxation and Stress Reduction Workbook" by Martha Davis, Elizabeth Robbins Eshelman, and Matthew McKay

- This workbook includes various meditation techniques alongside other methods for reducing stress.

Articles and Journals

1. "Mindfulness-Based Stress Reduction and Health Benefits: A Meta-Analysis" by Grossman, Niemann, Schmidt, and Walach

- Published in the Journal of Psychosomatic Research, this meta-analysis reviews the health benefits of mindfulness-based stress reduction (MBSR).

2. "Effects of Loving-Kindness Meditation on Emotions and Interpersonal Interactions" by Barbara L. Fredrickson, et al.

- Published in Journal of Personality and Social Psychology, this article examines the emotional and social benefits of loving-kindness meditation.

3. "The Impact of Meditation on Resting State Brain Networks" by Brewer, Worhunsky, Gray, et al.

- Published in Psychiatry Research: Neuroimaging, this study investigates how different meditation practices affect brain function and connectivity.

4. "Guided Imagery as a Therapeutic Tool in Medicine" by D. L. Gaynor

- Published in Alternative Therapies in Health and Medicine, this article explores the applications and benefits of guided imagery in medical settings.

Videos

1. "Mindfulness Meditation" (YouTube Channel)

- Offers a variety of guided mindfulness meditation sessions for different needs and durations.

- [Mindfulness Meditation](https://www.youtube.com/channel/UCwobzUc3z-0PrFpoRxNszXQ)

2. "The Honest Guys" (YouTube Channel)

- Provides guided meditations, including body scans and visualization techniques.

- [The Honest Guys](https://www.youtube.com/user/TheHonestGuys)

3. "Tara Brach" (YouTube Channel)

- Renowned meditation teacher Tara Brach offers guided meditations and talks on mindfulness and compassion.

- [Tara Brach](https://www.youtube.com/user/tarabrach)

Online Resources

1. Headspace

- A popular app offering guided meditations, mindfulness exercises, and courses on various meditation techniques.

- [Headspace](https://www.headspace.com)

2. Insight Timer

- A free app with a vast library of guided meditations, music tracks, and talks from meditation teachers worldwide.

- [Insight Timer](https://www.insighttimer.com)

3. Calm

- An app providing guided meditation sessions, sleep stories, and relaxation techniques for stress relief and better sleep.

- [Calm](https://www.calm.com)

4. Mindful.org

- A comprehensive resource for mindfulness and meditation, offering articles

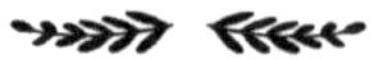

CHAPTER 4

CREATING A HOLISTIC STRESS RELIEF PLAN

*"To keep the body in good health is a duty...
otherwise we shall not be able to keep our mind
strong and clear." – Buddha*

Introduction

In today's fast-paced world, managing stress effectively requires a comprehensive approach that addresses both the mind and body. A holistic stress relief plan integrates various strategies, including yoga, meditation, healthy lifestyle choices, and mindful living practices. This chapter guides you through the process of creating a personalized plan to reduce stress and enhance overall well-being.

4.1 Assessing Your Stress Levels

The first step in creating a holistic stress relief plan is to assess your current stress levels. Understanding the sources and impacts of stress in your life helps tailor your approach to meet your specific needs.

Identifying Stressors

Begin by identifying the main stressors in your life. These can be related to work, relationships, financial concerns, health issues, or other personal challenges. Make a list of these stressors and consider their frequency and intensity.

Recognizing Symptoms of Stress

Next, recognize the symptoms of stress you experience. Common symptoms include headaches, muscle tension, fatigue, sleep disturbances, irritability, anxiety, and difficulty concentrating. Keeping a stress journal can help track these symptoms and their triggers.

Utilizing Stress Assessment Tools

Several tools and questionnaires are available to assess stress levels, such as the Perceived Stress Scale (PSS) and the Stress Symptom Checklist. These tools provide a more objective measure of your stress and can highlight areas needing the most attention.

Benefits of Assessing Stress Levels

Assessing your stress levels helps create a baseline to measure progress. It also brings awareness to how stress manifests in your life, guiding you in prioritizing areas for intervention. By understanding your stress profile, you can more effectively implement strategies that address your unique challenges.

4.2 Building a Personalized Yoga and Meditation Routine

Integrating yoga and meditation into your daily routine is a powerful way to manage stress. A personalized practice ensures that you engage in activities that resonate with you and fit your lifestyle.

Designing Your Yoga Practice

Choose yoga poses and sequences that address your specific needs and preferences. For beginners, simple poses like Child's Pose, Cat-Cow, and Downward-Facing Dog can be effective. As you advance, incorporate more complex poses and longer sequences. Aim for a balance of stretching, strengthening, and relaxation poses.

Incorporating Meditation Techniques

Select meditation techniques that complement your yoga practice and address your stress symptoms. Mindfulness meditation, focused attention meditation, and body scan meditation are all excellent choices. Start with short sessions of 5-10 minutes and gradually increase the duration as you become more comfortable.

Creating a Consistent Schedule

Consistency is key to reaping the benefits of yoga and meditation. Set a regular schedule for your practice, ideally at the same time each day. Morning practices can set a positive tone for the day, while evening sessions can help unwind and prepare for restful sleep.

Adapting to Your Needs

Remain flexible and open to adjusting your routine as needed. If certain poses or techniques do not feel right, explore alternatives. Listen to your body and mind, and make changes to ensure your practice remains enjoyable and effective.

4.3 Incorporating Healthy Lifestyle Choices

A holistic stress relief plan extends beyond yoga and meditation to include overall healthy lifestyle choices. These choices significantly impact your stress levels and overall well-being.

Nutrition and Hydration

Eating a balanced diet rich in fruits, vegetables, whole grains, lean proteins, and healthy fats supports your body's ability to cope with stress. Avoid excessive caffeine, sugar, and processed foods, which can exacerbate stress symptoms. Staying well-hydrated is also crucial for maintaining physical and mental health.

Regular Physical Activity

In addition to yoga, engage in regular physical activity such as walking, running, swimming, or strength training. Exercise releases endorphins, which are natural stress relievers. Aim for at least 30 minutes of moderate exercise most days of the week.

Adequate Sleep

Quality sleep is essential for stress management. Establish a regular sleep routine by going to bed and waking up at the same time each day. Create a relaxing bedtime ritual, avoid screens before bed, and ensure your sleep environment is comfortable and conducive to rest.

Social Connections

Maintaining healthy relationships and social connections provides emotional support and can significantly reduce stress. Spend time with loved ones, engage in community activities, and seek support from friends and family when needed.

Avoiding Unhealthy Coping Mechanisms

Avoid relying on unhealthy coping mechanisms such as smoking, excessive drinking, or overeating. These behaviors can temporarily alleviate stress but ultimately contribute to long-term health issues and increased stress levels.

4.4 Mindful Living and Daily Practices

Incorporating mindfulness into your daily life helps maintain a state of calm and awareness, reducing overall stress.

Practicing Mindfulness Throughout the Day

Bring mindfulness into everyday activities such as eating, walking, and even chores. Pay full attention to the present moment, engaging all your senses, and avoiding distractions. This practice can transform mundane tasks into opportunities for relaxation and presence.

Setting Intentions

Begin each day by setting positive intentions. Reflect on what you hope to achieve and how you want to approach your day. This simple practice can create a sense of purpose and direction, reducing stress and increasing motivation.

Taking Breaks

Regular breaks throughout the day are essential for maintaining productivity and reducing stress. Use these breaks to stretch, practice deep breathing, or take a short walk. Allowing yourself time to rest and recharge helps maintain focus and prevents burnout.

Gratitude Practice

Cultivating gratitude is a powerful way to shift focus from stressors to positive aspects of life. Keep a gratitude journal, noting things you are thankful for each day. This practice can enhance your mood, improve relationships, and increase overall well-being.

Digital Detox

In our technology-driven world, taking breaks from screens and digital devices is crucial for mental health. Set aside time each day to disconnect from digital media, reducing exposure to stressful news and social media. Use this time for mindfulness practices, reading, or engaging in hobbies.

4.5 Monitoring and Adjusting Your Plan

Creating a holistic stress relief plan is an ongoing process that requires regular monitoring and adjustments to ensure its effectiveness.

Tracking Progress

Keep a journal to track your stress levels, symptoms, and the effectiveness of your stress relief strategies. Note any changes in your physical and emotional state, as well as any external factors that may influence your stress.

Reflecting on Your Practice

Regularly reflect on your yoga, meditation, and lifestyle practices. Consider what is working well and what might need adjustment. Reflecting helps you stay engaged with your practice and make informed decisions about necessary changes.

Seeking Feedback

Seek feedback from trusted friends, family, or a professional mentor who can provide insights into your progress. They can offer valuable perspectives and suggestions for improving your stress relief plan.

Making Adjustments

Be open to making adjustments to your plan as needed. Life circumstances change, and what worked initially might need modification over time. Flexibility and willingness to adapt are key to maintaining an effective stress relief routine.

Professional Support

If you find it challenging to manage stress on your own, consider seeking support from a mental health professional. Therapists, counselors, and life coaches can provide guidance, tools, and techniques to enhance your stress management plan.

Conclusion

Creating a holistic stress relief plan involves a comprehensive approach that integrates yoga, meditation, healthy lifestyle choices, and mindful living practices. By assessing your stress levels, building a personalized routine, and incorporating mindful practices into daily life, you can effectively manage stress and enhance overall well-being. Regular monitoring and adjustments ensure that your plan remains effective and responsive to your evolving needs. With commitment and flexibility, a holistic approach can lead to a more balanced, peaceful, and fulfilling life.

Resources

Books

1. "The Miracle of Mindfulness" by Thích Nhất Hạnh

- A practical guide to mindfulness meditation, offering techniques and insights from a renowned Zen master.

2. "Wherever You Go, There You Are" by Jon Kabat-Zinn

- An accessible introduction to mindfulness meditation, emphasizing the practice of being present in everyday life.

3. "The Relaxation and Stress Reduction Workbook" by Martha Davis, Elizabeth Robbins Eshelman, and Matthew McKay

- This workbook includes various meditation techniques alongside other methods for reducing stress.

4. "Light on Yoga" by B.K.S. Iyengar

- A comprehensive guide to yoga poses and sequences, with detailed illustrations and instructions.

5. "The Yoga Sutras of Patanjali" translated by Sri Swami Satchidananda

- This ancient text is fundamental to understanding the philosophy and deeper aspects of yoga practice.

Articles and Journals

1. "Mindfulness-Based Stress Reduction and Health Benefits: A Meta-Analysis" by Grossman, Niemann, Schmidt, and Walach

- Published in the Journal of Psychosomatic Research, this meta-analysis reviews the health benefits of mindfulness-based stress reduction (MBSR).

2. "Effects of Loving-Kindness Meditation on Emotions and Interpersonal Interactions" by Barbara L. Fredrickson, et al.

- Published in Journal of Personality and Social Psychology, this article examines the emotional and social benefits of loving-kindness meditation.

3. "The Impact of Meditation on Resting State Brain Networks" by Brewer, Worhunsky, Gray, et al.

- Published in Psychiatry Research: Neuroimaging, this study investigates how different meditation practices affect brain function and connectivity.

4. "The Role of Physical Activity in Reducing Stress and Improving Mental Health" by Penedo and Dahn

- Published in Sports Medicine, this review highlights the benefits of physical activity for mental health and stress reduction

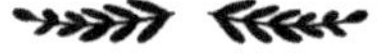

CHAPTER 5

ADVANCED YOGA AND MEDITATION PRACTICES

"Yoga is the journey of the self, through the self, to the self." – The Bhagavad Gita

Introduction

As you become more experienced in yoga and meditation, advancing your practice can lead to deeper levels of physical, mental, and spiritual well-being. This chapter explores advanced yoga poses, techniques for deepening meditation, and the synergy of combining both practices. It also delves into the benefits of yoga and meditation retreats and how technology can enhance your practice. By embracing these advanced practices, you can cultivate a more profound and transformative experience on your journey to holistic health.

5.1 Exploring Advanced Yoga Poses

Advanced yoga poses challenge your strength, flexibility, and balance, pushing the boundaries of your physical practice. These poses require a solid foundation in basic yoga asanas and a mindful approach to prevent injury.

Benefits of Advanced Yoga Poses

Advanced poses enhance physical strength, improve flexibility, and promote mental focus and discipline. They also encourage a deeper connection with the breath and body, fostering greater mindfulness and body awareness.

Examples of Advanced Poses

1. Headstand (Sirsasana)

- Known as the "king of asanas," headstand requires core strength, balance, and focus. Practice against a wall initially, and ensure proper alignment to avoid neck strain.

2. Forearm Stand (Pincha Mayurasana)

- This pose strengthens the shoulders, arms, and core. Use a wall for support as you build strength and confidence in balancing on your forearms.

3. Crow Pose (Bakasana)

- A challenging arm balance that strengthens the arms, wrists, and core. Focus on engaging your core and keeping your gaze forward to maintain balance.

4. Wheel Pose (Urdhva Dhanurasana)

- A deep backbend that opens the chest and shoulders while strengthening the legs and arms. Warm up thoroughly and progress slowly to avoid strain.

5. King Pigeon Pose (Eka Pada Rajakapotasana)

- A deep hip opener combined with a backbend, requiring flexibility in the hips, spine, and shoulders. Approach this pose gradually, using props as needed.

Tips for Practicing Advanced Poses

- Warm up thoroughly with foundational poses and stretches.

- Focus on alignment and use props to support your practice.

- Listen to your body and avoid pushing into pain.

- Practice regularly to build strength and flexibility.

- Seek guidance from experienced teachers or attend advanced yoga classes.

5.2 Deepening Your Meditation Practice

Deepening your meditation practice involves exploring advanced techniques, extending the duration of your sessions, and cultivating a deeper state of awareness and tranquility.

Techniques for Deepening Meditation

1. Vipassana Meditation

- An insight meditation that focuses on developing mindfulness and insight into the true nature of reality. It involves observing bodily sensations, thoughts, and emotions without attachment or aversion.

2. Transcendental Meditation (TM)

- A mantra-based meditation technique that promotes a deep state of restful alertness. Practitioners silently repeat a specific mantra to transcend ordinary thought and achieve a state of pure awareness.

3. Zen Meditation (Zazen)

- A seated meditation practice that emphasizes observing the breath and mind. It often involves counting breaths or practicing "shikantaza," or just sitting, with no specific focus.

4. Kundalini Meditation

- A practice aimed at awakening the dormant energy (Kundalini) at the base of the spine. It combines breath control, mantras, and physical postures to activate and channel this energy.

5. Loving-Kindness Meditation (Metta)

- A practice that cultivates unconditional love and compassion for oneself and others. It involves silently repeating phrases of goodwill and gradually expanding the circle of compassion.

Extending Meditation Duration

Gradually increase the duration of your meditation sessions to deepen your practice. Start with 5-10 minutes and gradually extend to 20-30 minutes or longer. Consistency is key, so aim to meditate at the same time each day.

Creating a Sacred Space

Create a dedicated meditation space that is quiet, comfortable, and free from distractions. Personalize it with items that inspire tranquility, such as candles, incense, or cushions. A sacred space enhances the meditative experience and signals to your mind that it is time for deep practice.

Mindful Living

Integrate mindfulness into all aspects of your life, not just during formal meditation sessions. Practice being fully present in everyday activities, such as eating, walking, and interacting with others. This holistic approach deepens your overall mindfulness and enriches your meditation practice.

5.3 Combining Yoga and Meditation

Combining yoga and meditation creates a synergistic practice that enhances the benefits of both disciplines. Yoga prepares the body and mind for meditation, while meditation deepens the mindfulness cultivated through yoga.

The Synergy of Yoga and Meditation

Yoga's physical postures (asanas) help release physical tension, making it easier to sit comfortably for meditation. The focus on breath and movement during yoga fosters a mindful awareness that carries over into meditation. Together, they create a holistic practice that addresses both physical and mental well-being.

Structuring a Combined Practice

1. Start with a Yoga Session

- Begin with a 20-30 minute yoga session to warm up the body and calm the mind. Focus on poses that release tension and promote relaxation.

2. Transition to Meditation

- After yoga, move directly into a meditation session. Sit comfortably and focus on your breath or chosen meditation technique. Start with 10-20 minutes of meditation and gradually extend the duration.

3. End with Relaxation

- Conclude your practice with a few minutes of relaxation in Corpse Pose (Savasana). Allow your body and mind to absorb the benefits of the combined practice.

Benefits of Combined Practice

- Enhanced relaxation and stress relief.

- Improved physical and mental flexibility.

- Greater awareness and mindfulness.

- A deeper connection between mind and body.

- Enhanced overall well-being and balance.

5.4 Yoga and Meditation Retreats

Attending a yoga and meditation retreat provides an immersive experience that deepens your practice and promotes profound relaxation and self-discovery.

Benefits of Retreats

Retreats offer a break from daily routines and stressors, allowing you to fully immerse yourself in practice. They provide an opportunity to learn from experienced teachers, connect with like-minded individuals, and explore new techniques in a supportive environment.

Types of Retreats

1. Silent Retreats

- Focus on meditation and mindfulness in a silent environment. These retreats often include guided meditations, mindful walking, and silent meals to promote deep inner reflection.

2. Yoga and Adventure Retreats

- Combine yoga practice with outdoor activities such as hiking, surfing, or skiing. These retreats offer a balance of physical activity and relaxation, set in scenic locations.

3. Detox Retreats

- Focus on cleansing and rejuvenating the body through yoga, meditation, and a detoxifying diet. These retreats often include workshops on nutrition and healthy living.

4. Spiritual Retreats

- Emphasize spiritual growth and self-discovery through yoga, meditation, and spiritual teachings. These retreats may include workshops on philosophy, self-inquiry, and personal development.

Preparing for a Retreat

- Research and choose a retreat that aligns with your goals and interests.

- Prepare physically and mentally for the retreat experience.

- Pack comfortable clothing, a yoga mat, and any personal items that support your practice.

- Approach the retreat with an open mind and willingness to fully engage in the experience.

5.5 Using Technology to Enhance Practice

Technology offers various tools and resources to support and enhance your yoga and meditation practice, making it more accessible and engaging.

Yoga Apps and Online Classes

- YogaGlo

- Offers a wide range of online yoga classes for all levels, taught by experienced instructors. Classes can be streamed or downloaded for offline practice.

- Alo Moves

- Provides access to thousands of yoga, fitness, and mindfulness classes. The platform offers structured programs and workshops to deepen your practice.

- Down Dog

- A customizable yoga app that generates unique yoga sequences based on your preferences, skill level, and available time.

Meditation Apps

- Headspace

- Offers guided meditations, mindfulness exercises, and courses on various meditation techniques. The app includes programs for beginners and advanced practitioners.

- Calm

- Provides guided meditation sessions, sleep stories, and relaxation techniques. The app also features music and soundscapes to enhance meditation.

- Insight Timer

- A free app with a vast library of guided meditations, music tracks, and talks from meditation teachers worldwide.

Wearable Technology

- Fitness Trackers

- Devices like Fitbit and Apple Watch monitor physical activity, heart rate, and sleep patterns. They can help track progress and ensure a balanced lifestyle.

- Meditation Headbands

- Devices like Muse provide real-time feedback on brain activity during meditation. They help improve focus and deepen meditation practice by guiding users through sessions based on their brainwave activity.

Virtual Reality

- VR Meditation Apps

- Virtual reality apps such as TRIPP and Guided Meditation VR offer immersive meditation experiences, transporting users to calming environments and guiding them through meditation practices.

Benefits of Using Technology

- Accessibility to a wide range of classes and resources.

- Ability to practice at your own pace and convenience.

- Personalized guidance and feedback.

- Enhanced motivation and engagement.

- Support in tracking progress and maintaining consistency.

Conclusion

Advancing your yoga and meditation practice opens up new dimensions of physical, mental, and spiritual well-being. By exploring advanced poses, deepening your meditation techniques, and combining both practices, you can experience profound personal growth and stress relief

Resources

Books

1. "Light on Yoga" by B.K.S. Iyengar - Comprehensive guide to yoga poses and sequences.

2. "The Heart of Yoga" by T.K.V. Desikachar - Guide to developing a personalized yoga and meditation practice.

3. "The Art of Meditation" by Matthieu Ricard - Insights into various meditation techniques.

4. "Waking Up" by Sam Harris - Practical advice on meditation from a secular perspective.

5. "The Power of Now" by Eckhart Tolle - Emphasizes the importance of living in the present moment.

Articles and Journals

1. "The Impact of Yoga on Physical and Mental Health" - Review of yoga's benefits, published in Complementary Therapies in Medicine.

2. "Mindfulness Meditation: A Research-Proven Way to Reduce Stress" - Overview of mindfulness meditation by Harvard Health Publishing.

3. "Yoga-Based Interventions in Mental Health" - Review of yoga's effectiveness, published in Frontiers in Psychiatry.

4. "Transcendental Meditation and Improved Academic Performance" - Study published in Education.

5. "Zen Meditation and Neuroscience" - Examines Zen meditation's effects, published in Cognitive Processing.

Websites and Online Resources

1. Yoga Journal (www.yogajournal.com) - Information on advanced yoga poses and sequences.

2. Headspace (www.headspace.com) - Guided meditations and mindfulness resources.

3. Insight Timer (www.insighttimer.com) - Free app with a vast library of guided meditations.

4. YogaGlo (www.yogaglo.com) - Online yoga classes, including advanced sequences.

5. Calm (www.calm.com) - Guided meditation sessions and relaxation techniques.

Retreat Centers

1. Kripalu Center for Yoga & Health (www.kripalu.org) - Various yoga and meditation retreats.

2. Spirit Rock Meditation Center (www.spiritrock.org) - Meditation retreats focusing on mindfulness and loving-kindness.

3. Omega Institute (www.eomega.org) - Yoga and meditation retreats and workshops.

4. Esalen Institute (www.esalen.org) - Workshops on advanced yoga and meditation.

5. Sivananda Ashram Yoga Retreat (www.sivanandabahamas.org) - Immersive yoga and meditation retreats.

Apps and Technology

1. Alo Moves (www.alomoves.com) - Yoga, fitness, and mindfulness classes.

2. Down Dog (www.downdogapp.com) - Customizable yoga sequences.

3. Muse (www.choosemuse.com) - Meditation headband with real-time feedback.

4. TRIPP (www.tripp.com) - Virtual reality meditation experiences.

5. Guided Meditation VR (www.guidedmeditationvr.com) - Guided meditation in virtual environments.

CHAPTER 6

LONG-TERM STRESS RELIEF STRATEGIES

"The greatest weapon against stress is our ability to choose one thought over another." – William James

Introduction

In the journey towards a balanced and stress-free life, consistency and adaptability are key. This chapter delves into strategies for maintaining long-term stress relief through sustained practice, adaptability, teaching, exploring complementary therapies, and cultivating a holistic approach to living. By integrating these strategies into your daily routine, you can create a resilient foundation for managing stress effectively.

6.1 Maintaining Consistency in Practice

Consistency is crucial in reaping the long-term benefits of yoga and meditation. Regular practice helps embed these techniques into your lifestyle, making them second nature.

Establishing a Routine

- Set a Schedule: Dedicate specific times each day for yoga and meditation. Morning sessions can invigorate your day, while evening sessions can help you unwind.

- Create a Dedicated Space: Designate a quiet, comfortable space for practice. A consistent environment fosters a habit.

- Start Small: Begin with manageable sessions (e.g., 10-15 minutes) and gradually increase the duration.

Staying Motivated

- Set Goals: Establish clear, achievable goals for your practice. Whether it's mastering a new pose or meditating for longer periods, goals keep you focused.

- Track Progress: Keep a journal to record your experiences, challenges, and improvements.

- Join a Community: Engage with like-minded individuals through yoga classes or meditation groups. Community support can enhance motivation.

Overcoming Obstacles

- Be Flexible: Adapt your practice to fit your schedule. Shorter, more frequent sessions can be just as effective as longer ones.

- Forgive Yourself: Missed a session? Don't dwell on it. Return to your routine with renewed commitment.

6.2 Adapting to Life Changes

Life changes, such as a new job, relocation, or family dynamics, can disrupt your practice. Adapting to these changes ensures continued stress relief.

Integrating Practice into New Routines

- Adjust Your Schedule: Find new times that work better with your current lifestyle. Early morning or late evening can be quieter, more private times.

- Use Technology: Online classes and apps can provide flexibility and guidance when you can't attend in-person sessions.

Remaining Flexible

- Modify Practices: Adapt yoga poses and meditation techniques to suit your current physical and mental state. Gentle yoga or shorter meditation sessions may be more feasible during stressful times.

- Stay Connected: Maintain communication with your yoga and meditation community. They can provide support and motivation during transitions.

6.3 Teaching Yoga and Meditation

Teaching yoga and meditation can deepen your own practice and share the benefits with others.

Benefits of Teaching

- Deeper Understanding: Teaching requires a thorough understanding of techniques and principles, enhancing your own practice.

- Community Building: Creates a supportive network and fosters connections with like-minded individuals.

- Personal Growth: Teaching challenges you to grow personally and professionally.

Getting Started

- Certification: Enroll in accredited teacher training programs. Certifications add credibility and ensure comprehensive knowledge.

- Practice Teaching: Start with friends, family, or small groups to build confidence and gain experience.

- Continuous Learning: Attend workshops, read extensively, and engage with other teachers to keep your knowledge fresh and updated.

6.4 Exploring Other Complementary Therapies

Complementary therapies can enhance the benefits of yoga and meditation, offering additional tools for stress relief.

Types of Complementary Therapies

1. Acupuncture: Involves inserting thin needles into specific points on the body to balance energy and reduce stress.

2. Massage Therapy: Helps relax muscles, improve circulation, and reduce stress hormones.

3. Aromatherapy: Uses essential oils to promote relaxation and improve mood.

4. Tai Chi and Qigong: Gentle, flowing movements combined with breath control to enhance relaxation and mindfulness.

5. Herbal Remedies: Natural supplements like chamomile, valerian root, and ashwagandha can support stress management.

Integrating Complementary Therapies

- Consult Professionals: Seek advice from certified practitioners to ensure safe and effective integration of therapies.

- Personalize Your Approach: Experiment with different therapies to find what works best for you.

- Consistency is Key: Regularly incorporate chosen therapies into your routine for maximum benefit.

6.5 Living a Balanced, Stress-Free Life

Achieving long-term stress relief requires a holistic approach to lifestyle. Balance and mindfulness are essential components.

Cultivating Mindfulness

- Mindful Eating: Pay attention to the taste, texture, and sensation of each bite. Avoid distractions during meals.

- Mindful Movement: Incorporate mindfulness into daily activities like walking, cleaning, or driving.

- Gratitude Practice: Regularly reflect on what you are grateful for. This shifts focus from stressors to positive aspects of life.

Work-Life Balance

- Set Boundaries: Establish clear boundaries between work and personal life. Avoid checking work emails outside of office hours.

- Prioritize Self-Care: Schedule regular time for activities that rejuvenate you, such as hobbies, socializing, or relaxation.

Creating a Support System

- Seek Social Support: Build a network of friends, family, and professionals who support your well-being.

- Professional Help: Don't hesitate to seek help from mental health professionals if stress becomes overwhelming.

Continuous Self-Reflection

- Regular Check-Ins: Periodically assess your stress levels and overall well-being. Adjust your routines and practices as needed.

- Celebrate Progress: Acknowledge and celebrate your achievements and improvements in managing stress.

Conclusion

Long-term stress relief is a journey that requires consistency, adaptability, and a holistic approach to living. By maintaining regular practice, adapting to life changes, teaching, exploring complementary therapies, and striving for a balanced life, you can achieve enduring peace and well-being. Remember, the goal is not to eliminate stress entirely but to develop resilience and a toolkit of strategies to manage it effectively.

Resources

Books

1. "The Miracle of Mindfulness" by Thich Nhat Hanh - A guide to incorporating mindfulness into daily life.

2. "The Yoga Bible" by Christina Brown - A comprehensive guide to yoga poses and practices.

3. "The Meditation Bible" by Madonna Gauding - Techniques and practices for various forms of meditation.

4. "The Healing Power of Mindfulness" by Jon Kabat-Zinn - Insights on mindfulness-based stress reduction.

5. "The Body Keeps the Score" by Bessel van der Kolk - Explores how trauma and stress impact the body and mind.

Articles and Journals

1. "Long-Term Benefits of Yoga and Meditation" by Catherine Woodyard - Published in The Journal of Alternative and Complementary Medicine.

2. "Adaptation to Life Changes Through Mindfulness" by Michael Baime - Published in Current Opinion in Psychiatry.

3. "Teaching Mindfulness: A Practical Guide for Clinicians and Educators" by Donald McCown, Diane Reibel, and Marc S. Micozzi - Comprehensive resource on teaching mindfulness.

4. "Complementary Therapies for Stress Management" by Mary L. Hardy - Published in Cochrane Database of Systematic Reviews.

5. "Balancing Work and Life: Practical Strategies" by Jeff Davidson - Published in Journal of Business Research.

Websites and Online Resources

1. Mindful (www.mindful.org) - Articles and resources on mindfulness and meditation.

2. Yoga Alliance (www.yogaalliance.org) - Information on yoga teacher training and certification.

3. National Center for Complementary and Integrative Health (www.nccih.nih.gov) - Research and resources on complementary therapies.

4. Headspace (www.headspace.com) - Guided meditations and mindfulness resources.

5. Calm (www.calm.com) - Meditation and relaxation techniques.

May I Ask You For A Small Favor?

I want to express my sincere gratitude for choosing to invest your time in reading this book. Your decision to explore this work among countless others means a lot to me.

I hope that within these pages, you've discovered actionable insights that can enhance your daily life. Your journey doesn't have to end here, though.

May I kindly request an additional 30 seconds of your valuable time?

Sharing your thoughts about the book through a review would be immensely appreciated. Your review serves as a beacon, guiding other readers to take a chance on my books. It's a small gesture that carries significant weight in the world of authors.

To submit your review effortlessly, please click on the link below. It will take you directly to the book's review page:

"Yoga and Meditation for Stress Relief"

Alternatively, you can also find the "**Reviews Section**" of this book's page on Amazon.

Your review will require just a minute of your time but will make a monumental difference in helping me connect with a broader audience and I eagerly look forward to reading your review.

Once again, thank you for your unwavering support of my work.

DISCLAIMER

This book is for educational purposes only. Readers acknowledge that the author does not render legal, financial, medical, or professional advice. The content within this book has been derived from various sources. Please consult a licensed professional before attempting any techniques outlined in this book.

By reading this document, the reader agrees that under no circumstances is the author responsible for any direct or indirect losses incurred as a result of the use of the information contained within this document, including but not limited to errors, omissions, or inaccuracies.

Adherence to all applicable laws and regulations, including international, federal, state, and local governing professional licensing, business practices, advertising, and all other jurisdictions, is the sole responsibility of the purchaser or reader.

Neither the author nor the publisher assumes any responsibility or liability whatsoever on behalf of the purchaser or reader of these materials. Any perceived slight of any individual or organization is purely unintentional.

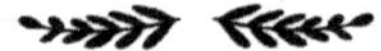

www.ingramcontent.com/pod-product-compliance
Lightning Source LLC
Chambersburg PA
CBHW051757250726

48659CB00001B/470